PILATES FOR SENIORS

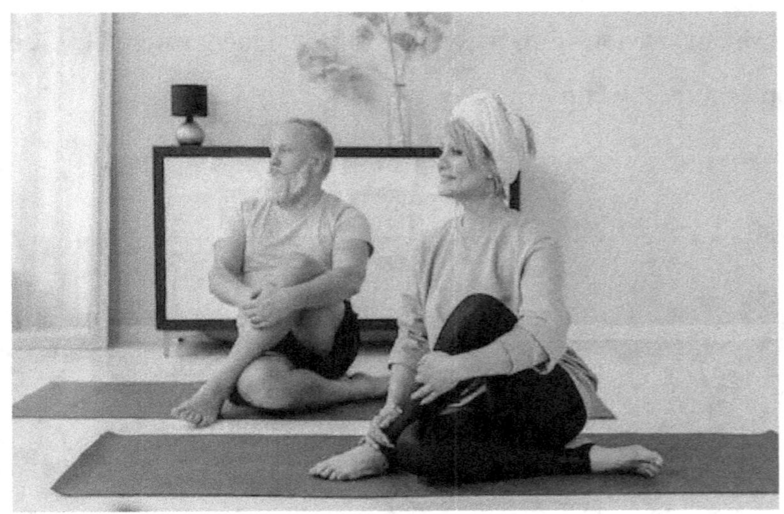

Dr. Kimberly Carlos

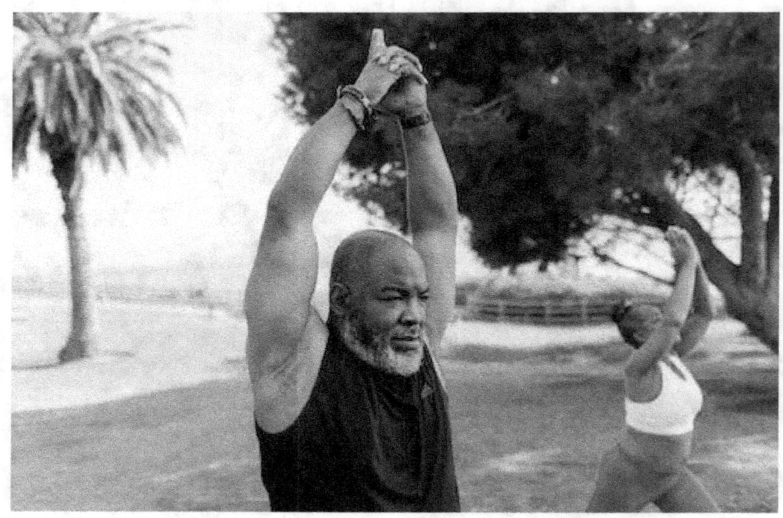

TABLE OF CONTENT

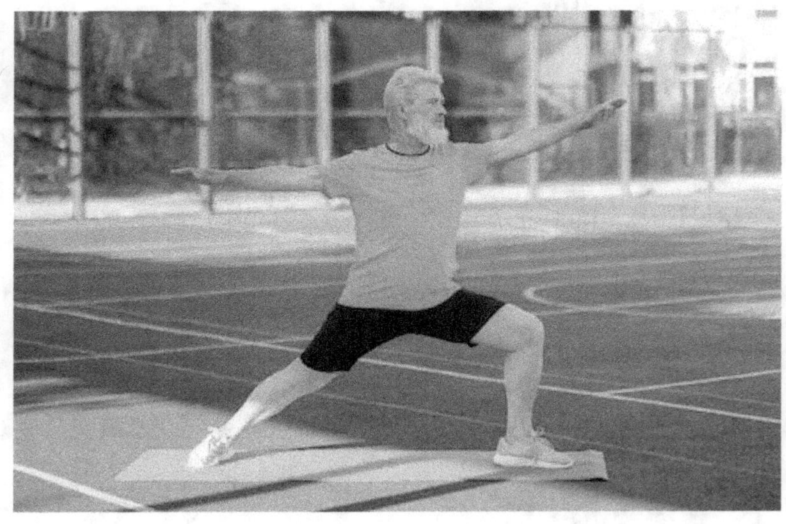

INTRODUCTION

Once upon a time in the peaceful town of Harmony Grove, there lived a compassionate and lively woman named Emily. Emily had a passion for fitness and a heartwarming desire to help others, especially seniors, lead healthier and happier lives. With this vision in mind, she decided to open a special Pilates studio tailored exclusively for seniors.

Emily's Pilates for Seniors quickly became the talk of the town. The studio was adorned with vibrant colors, cozy chairs, and gentle music, creating a warm and inviting atmosphere for the elderly residents.

Emily understood that many seniors were hesitant to engage in physical activities due to fear of injury or simply feeling out of place in conventional gyms. Hence, she designed her classes to be gentle, adaptive, and personalized to meet each senior's unique needs.

Word about Emily's Pilates for Seniors spread like wildfire, and soon enough, the studio was bustling with eager participants.

From the sprightly octogenarians to the more reserved retirees, Emily welcomed them all with open arms. She focused on building a sense of community within the studio, where everyone felt comfortable and supported.

One of her most enthusiastic students was Mr. Lawrence, an 80-year-old retired professor. He initially joined the classes with trepidation, unsure if he could keep up. But Emily's patience and encouragement soon put him at ease. With every session, he grew stronger and more flexible, surprising himself and his family with his newfound vitality.

Another regular was Mrs. Thompson, a 75-year-old widow who had been feeling lonely and isolated since her husband's passing. The Pilates classes not only improved her physical health but also lifted her spirits. She found companionship and friendship among the other seniors, and they often gathered after class for tea and lively conversations.

Through her Pilates classes, Emily witnessed inspiring transformations. Seniors who had once struggled to walk without assistance were now moving with grace and confidence. Aches and pains diminished, replaced by smiles and laughter.

It was a sight that filled Emily's heart with joy and pride.

As the studio thrived, Emily's dedication and love for her senior students shone through. She organized special outings, picnics, and even charity events to give back to the community that had embraced her with open arms.

Emily's Pilates for Seniors became much more than just a fitness studio; it became a haven for the elderly, a place where they could feel valued, supported, and cared for. Emily's legacy continued to grow as more and more seniors experienced the positive impact of her gentle approach to Pilates.

And so, in the little town of Harmony Grove, Emily's Pilates for Seniors became a heartwarming tale of how one woman's passion and empathy transformed the lives of many, inspiring them to embrace their golden years with renewed vigor and happiness.

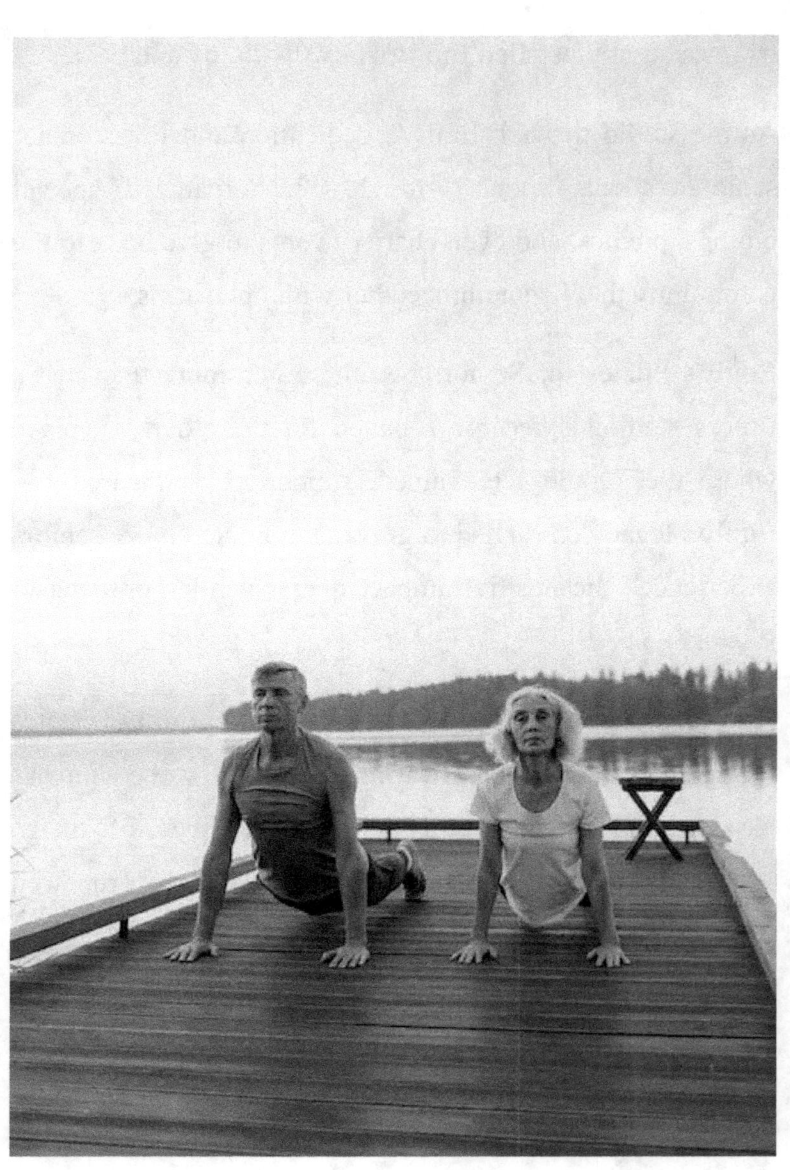

CHAPTER ONE

Pilate for Seniors Benefits

As we age, staying active becomes increasingly important for maintaining overall health and well-being. While high-impact workouts might not be suitable for everyone, Pilates offers an excellent alternative, especially for seniors. Pilates is a low-impact exercise system that focuses on core strength, flexibility, balance, and body awareness.

It provides numerous benefits for seniors, both physically and mentally, making it an ideal fitness option for this age group. In this book, we will explore the advantages of Pilates for seniors and provide a step-by-step guide on how to follow a Pilates routine tailored to their needs.

Benefits of Pilates for Seniors:

1. Improved Core Strength: Pilates places significant emphasis on the core muscles, which support the spine and contribute to overall stability. Strengthening the core can help seniors maintain proper posture and reduce the risk of back pain.

2. Enhanced Flexibility: As we age, our muscles tend to stiffen, leading to reduced flexibility. Pilates incorporates a range of stretching exercises that promote suppleness and help seniors maintain a full range of motion.

3. Better Balance and Coordination: Pilates exercises often involve performing movements while balancing on unstable surfaces, which helps improve balance and coordination. This is especially beneficial for seniors who are prone to falls.

4. Joint Health: The controlled and gentle movements in Pilates are easy on the joints, making it an ideal exercise for seniors with arthritis or other joint issues.

5. Increased Bone Density: Weight-bearing exercises, like certain Pilates movements, can help increase bone density, reducing the risk of osteoporosis.

6. Stress Reduction: Pilates promotes mind-body awareness, encouraging seniors to focus on their breath and movements. This mindfulness aspect can help reduce stress and improve mental well-being.

7. Social Interaction: Participating in group Pilates classes provides an opportunity for seniors to socialize, which is essential for mental and emotional health.

Getting Started with Pilates for Seniors:

Before beginning any exercise program, it's essential for seniors to consult their healthcare provider, especially if they have any pre-existing medical conditions or concerns**1. Find a Qualified Instructor:** Look for a Pilates instructor who specializes in working with seniors or offers classes tailored to their needs. A skilled instructor will ensure that seniors perform exercises correctly and safely.

2. Start with Basic Exercises: Beginners should start with foundational Pilates exercises that focus on breathing, core activation, and gentle movements. These exercises build a solid base for more advanced movements.

3. Use Props for Support: Props like a Pilates ball or resistance bands can provide additional support during exercises and allow seniors to gradually build strength and flexibility.

4. Listen to Your Body: Seniors should never push themselves beyond their comfort level. If an exercise feels too challenging, they can modify it or ask the instructor for an alternative.

5. Consistency is Key: To experience the full benefits of Pilates, consistency is essential. Seniors should aim for regular practice, even if it's just a few times a week.

6. Stay Hydrated: Seniors should drink plenty of water before, during, and after Pilates sessions to stay hydrated.

7. Warm-Up and Cool Down: It's crucial for seniors to warm up before starting Pilates exercises and cool down afterward to prevent injury and improve flexibility.

Pilates is a wonderful fitness option for seniors looking to enhance their physical and mental well-being. With its focus on gentle, controlled movements, Pilates offers numerous benefits, including improved core strength, flexibility, balance, and reduced stress. By finding a qualified instructor and following a routine tailored to their needs, seniors can embark on a fulfilling Pilates journey that will contribute to a healthier and happier life.

CHAPTER TWO

14-Day Pilates for Seniors Meal Plan

DAY 1

- Breakfast: Scrambled eggs with spinach and tomatoes, whole-grain toast, and a glass of orange juice.
- Lunch: Mixed greens, cucumber, cherry tomatoes, and grilled chicken salad with a mild vinaigrette dressing.
- Snack: Greek yogurt with mixed berries and a drizzle of honey.
- Dinner: fish baked in the oven with quinoa and steam broccoli.

DAY 2

- Breakfast: Oatmeal with sliced bananas and a sprinkle of walnuts.
- Lunch: Turkey and avocado wrap with whole-grain tortilla and a side of carrot sticks.
- Snack: Sliced apple with almond butter.
- Dinner: Stir-fried tofu with bell peppers, snap peas, and brown rice.

DAY 3

- Breakfast: Whole-grain waffles with Greek yogurt and fresh strawberries.
- Lunch: Lentil and vegetable soup with a whole-grain roll.
- Snack: Celery sticks with hummus.
- Dinner: Grilled chicken breast with sweet potato mash and asparagus.

DAY 4

- Breakfast: omelet with mushrooms and spinach and whole-grain bread.
- Lunch: feta cheese and roasted veggie quinoa salad.
- Snack: Handful of mixed nuts.
- Dinner: Baked cod with lemon-dill sauce, steamed green beans, and quinoa.

DAY 5

- Breakfast: spinach, banana, almond milk, and chia seed smoothie.
- Lunch: Chickpea and cucumber salad with a light lemon-tahini dressing.
- Snack: Sliced pear with cottage cheese.
- Dinner: Grilled shrimp with marinara sauce and zucchini noodles.

DAY 6

- Breakfast: parfait of yogurt, granola, and berries.
- Lunch: Spinach and feta stuffed chicken breast with roasted sweet potatoes.
- Snack: Carrot and cucumber sticks with tzatziki sauce.
- Dinner: Baked tilapia with mango salsa and quinoa.

DAY 7

- Breakfast: Whole-grain pancakes with fresh blueberries and a dollop of Greek yogurt.
- Lunch: Fresh mozzarella, cherry tomatoes, and basil leaves in a caprese salad.
- Snack: Sliced peaches with cottage cheese.
- Dinner: Vegetable stir-fry with tofu and brown rice.

DAY 8

- Breakfast: Scrambled eggs with diced peppers and onions, served with whole-grain toast.
- Lunch: Mediterranean chickpea salad with cucumber, red onion, olives, and feta cheese.
- Snack: Sliced cucumber with a sprinkle of Tajin seasoning.

-   Dinner: Baked chicken thighs with sweet potato fries
    and steamed broccoli.

DAY 9

-   Breakfast: Smoothie bowl with banana, mango, and
    a handful of almonds.
-   Lunch: Turkey and avocado lettuce wraps with a side
    of cherry tomatoes.
-   Snack: Sliced kiwi with a drizzle of honey.
-   Dinner: Grilled vegetable skewers with herbed
    quinoa.

DAY 10

-   Breakfast: Greek yogurt with honey, walnuts, and a
    mix of fresh berries.
-   Lunch: Portobello mushroom stuffed with spinach
    and feta served with mixed greens on the side.
-   Snack: Sliced bell peppers with hummus.
-   Dinner: Baked cod with lemon-butter sauce, roasted
    Brussels sprouts, and wild rice.

DAY 11

- Breakfast: Whole-grain waffles with a dollop of Greek yogurt and sliced strawberries.
- Lunch: Lentil soup with a whole-grain roll.
- Snack: a little amount of trail mix with nuts and dried fruits.
- Dinner: Grilled chicken breast with sweet potato mash and steamed green beans.

DAY 12

- Breakfast: Veggie omelet with mushrooms, tomatoes, and spinach, served with whole-grain toast.
- Lunch: Quinoa salad with roasted vegetables and goat cheese.
- Snack: Sliced apple with almond butter.
- Dinner: Baked salmon with dill sauce, asparagus, and quinoa.

DAY 13

- Breakfast: spinach, banana, almond milk, and chia seed smoothie.
- Lunch: Chickpea and cucumber salad with a light lemon-tahini dressing.
- Snack: Sliced pear with cottage cheese.
- Dinner: Grilled shrimp with marinara sauce and zucchini noodles.

DAY 14

- Breakfast: parfait of yogurt, granola, and berries.
- Lunch: Roasted sweet potatoes and chicken breast filled with spinach and feta.
- Snack: Carrot and cucumber sticks with tzatziki sauce.
- Dinner: Baked tilapia with mango salsa and quinoa.

General Tips

1. Stay hydrated by drinking plenty of water throughout the day.

2. Opt for whole grains, lean proteins, and a variety of fruits and vegetables.

3. Limit processed foods, sugary drinks, and high-sodium snacks.

4. Practice portion control to prevent overeating.

5. Enjoy meals mindfully, savoring each bite and eating slowly.

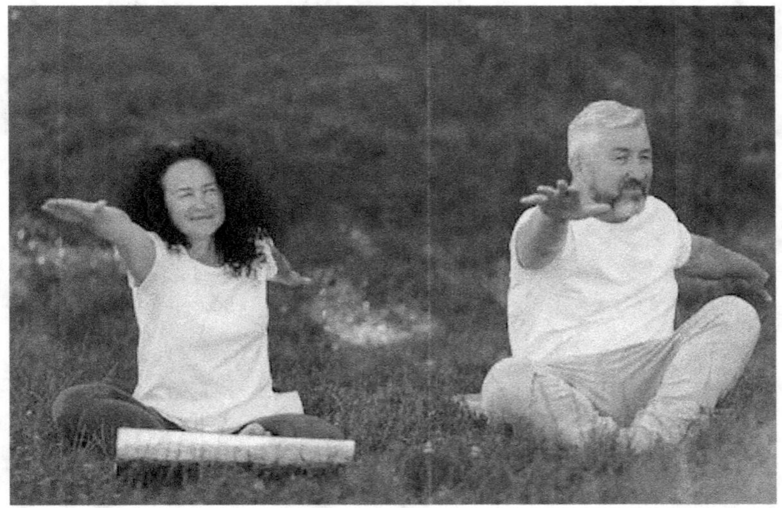

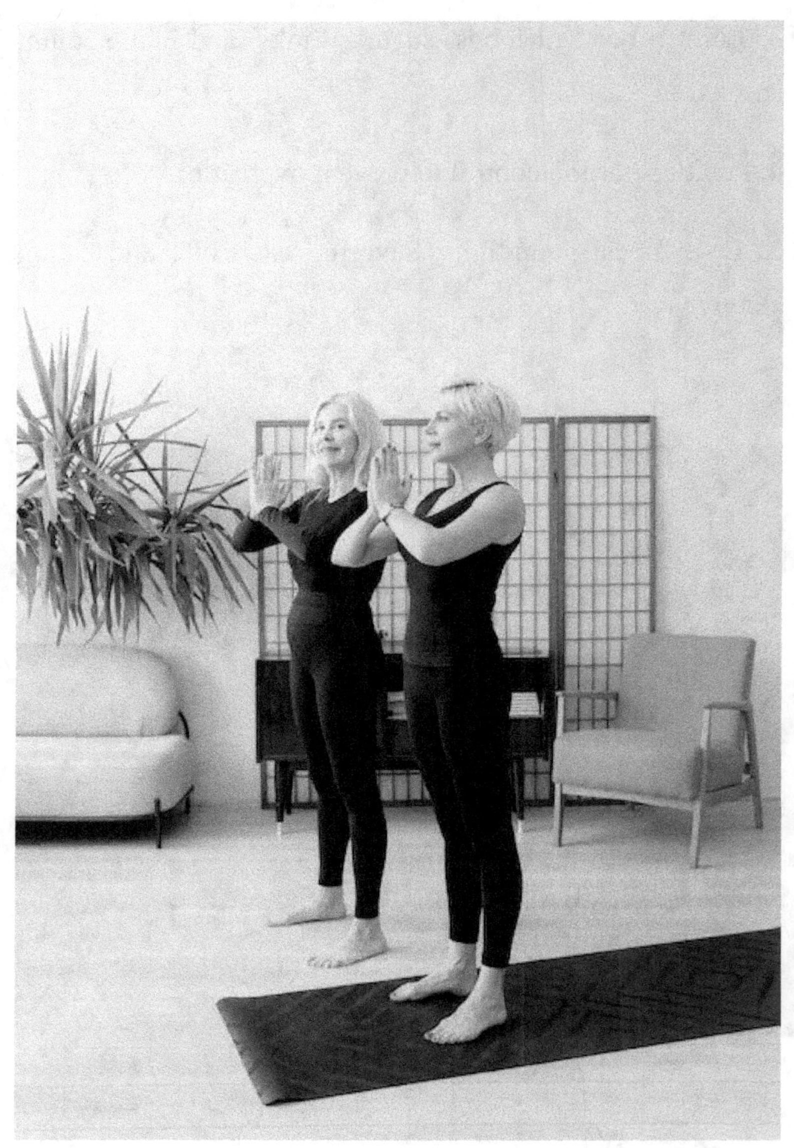

CHAPTER THREE

Pilate for Senior Exercises and How to Do Them

1. Breathing Exercise

- Maintain a neutral posture as you sit or lie down.
- Inhale deeply through the nose, expanding the lungs.
- Exhale slowly and completely through the mouth, engaging the core.

2. Pelvic Tilt

- Lie on your back with your feet flat on the ground and your knees bent.
- Breathe in to get ready, exhale, and tilt your pelvis slightly forward while contracting your abs.
- Inhale, then exhale to return to your starting position.

3. Leg Slides

- Lie on your back with one leg extended and one knee bent.
- While keeping your spine neutral, slid the extended leg along the floor toward your chest.
- Return the leg to its starting position by sliding it.

4. Pelvic Clock

- Lie on your back with your feet flat on the ground and your knees bent.

- Imagine a clock face over your pelvis. Tilt the pelvis to each number on the clock, exploring the range of motion.

5. Heel Slides

- Lie on your back with your feet flat on the ground and your knees bent.

- Slide one heel along the floor, extending the leg fully.

- Slide the heel back to the starting position and repeat with the other leg.

6. Arm Circles

- Sit or stand with arms extended out to the sides.
- Circle the arms forward in a controlled motion, then reverse the direction.

7. Knee Folds

- Take a seat in a chair with your feet flat on the ground.
- While clutching it with both hands, lift one leg toward your chest.
- Repeat on the other side after releasing the leg.

8. Shoulder Bridge

- Lie on your back with your feet flat on the ground and your knees bent.
- Raise your hips off the floor so that your body forms a bridge.
- Bringing the hips back to the ground.

9. Arm Raises

- Arms by sides while you stand or sit.
- Exhale to bring the arms back down after raising them aloft.

10. Side Leg Lifts

- Legs outstretched, lie on your side.
- Lift the top leg towards the ceiling, then lower it back down.
- Repeat on the other side.

11. Neck Nods

- Straighten your spine when you stand or sit.
- Gently nod your head forward, tucking the chin, then lift it back up to the starting position.

12. Spine Stretch

- Sit tall with legs extended and feet flexed.

- Inhale to lengthen the spine, then exhale and hinge forward from the hips, reaching towards your toes.

13. Arm Pulls

- Sit with your feet contracted and your legs extended.

- Reach the arms forward, then pull them back towards your hips, engaging the upper back.

14. Clamshells

- Lie on your side with your feet together and your knees bent.

- Lift the top knee while keeping the feet together, then lower it back down.

- Repeat on the other side.

15. Cat-Cow Stretch

- Position yourself on your hands and knees.

- Inhale to arch the back and lift the head (Cow), then exhale to round the back and tuck the chin (Cat).

16. Arm Circles in Quadruped

- Get down on your hands and knees in a tabletop position to begin.
- Circle one arm forward and then backward, maintaining stability in the core.
- Repeat with the other arm.

17. Leg Circles

- Lie on your back with your extended leg pointed upward.
- Circle the extended leg, keeping the hips stable and the core engaged.
- Reverse the direction of the circle.

18. Seated Twist

- Sit up straight with your legs out in front of you.
- Twist your torso to one side, placing your opposite hand on the floor behind you for support.
- Repeat on the other side.

19. Chest Opener

- Place your hands behind your back when standing or sitting.
- Inhale to lift the chest and open the shoulders, then exhale to release.

20. Side Bend

- Sit tall with legs extended to one side.
- Reach the arm overhead and stretch towards the opposite side.
- Repeat on the other side.

21. Mermaid Stretch

- Sit with one leg bent and the other extended to the side.
- Reach the arm overhead and bend sideways towards the extended leg.
- Repeat on the other side.

22. Single Leg Circles

- Lie on your back with your extended leg pointed upward.
- Circle the extended leg in a controlled motion, keeping the hips stable.
- Reverse the direction of the circle.

23. Arm Reach and Roll

- Sit tall with legs extended and arms forward.

- Inhale to reach the arms overhead, then exhale to roll the spine down one vertebra at a time.

- Take a breath in to rise back to the beginning position.

24. Seated Marching

- Take a seat in a chair with your feet flat on the ground.

- One knee should be raised to your chest and then brought back down.

- Repeat with the other leg.

25. Ankle Circles

- Sit on a chair with feet lifted off the floor.

- Circle one ankle in a clockwise motion, then reverse the direction.

- Repeat with the other ankle.

26. Chest Lift

- Lie on your back with your feet flat on the ground and your knees bent.
- Lift your shoulders, neck, and head off the floor while contracting your abs.
- Retract your steps to the beginning point.

27. Side Stretch

- Sit tall with legs extended to one side.
- Reach one arm overhead and stretch to the opposite side.
- Repeat on the other side.

28. Hip Abduction with Resistance Band

- Wrap your ankles in a resistance band.
- Stand tall and lift one leg sideways against the resistance of the band.
- Repeat with the other leg.

29. Wrist Rolls

- Sit or stand with arms extended forward.
- Roll the wrists in circular motions, first in one direction, then the other.

30. Seated Spinal Twist

- Sit tall with legs extended.

- Twist your torso to one side while supporting yourself with your hands behind you and one hand on the knee to the opposite.

- Repeat on the other side.

31. Seated Leg Circles

- Sit tall with legs extended and feet flexed.

- Circle one leg in a controlled motion, keeping the hips stable.

- Reverse the direction of the circle.

32. Side Leg Lifts with Resistance Band

- Wrap your ankles in a resistance band.
- Stand tall and lift one leg sideways against the resistance of the band.
- Repeat with the other leg.

33. Seated Row

- Sit tall with a resistance band wrapped around your feet and hold the ends of the band with both hands.
- Pull the band towards your torso, engaging the upper back.
- Release and repeat.

34. Seated Forward Bend

- Sit up straight with your legs out in front of you.
- Inhale to lengthen the spine, then exhale and hinge forward from the hips, reaching towards your toes.

35. Bridge with Leg Lift

- Lie on your back with your feet flat on the ground and your knees bent.
- Lift your hips off the floor, then extend one leg towards the ceiling.
- Lower the leg and lower your hips back down to the floor.
- Repeat with the other leg.

36. Leg Press

- Take a seat in a chair with your feet flat on the ground.
- Press one foot forward, extending the leg, then release back to the starting position.
- Repeat with the other leg.

37. Seated Chest Opener

- Sit tall with hands clasped behind your back.

- Inhale to lift the chest and open the shoulders, then exhale to release.

38. Side Bend with Resistance Band

- Stand tall with a resistance band looped over your head and under one foot.

- Reach the arm overhead and bend sideways towards the opposite side.

- Repeat on the other side.

39. Standing Hip Extension

- Stand tall with hands resting on a chair for support.

- Lift one leg backward, extending the hip, then lower it back down.

- Repeat with the other leg.

40. Chest Expansion with Resistance Band

- Stand tall with a resistance band held in front of you at chest height.

- Open your arms wide, stretching the band, then release back to the starting position.

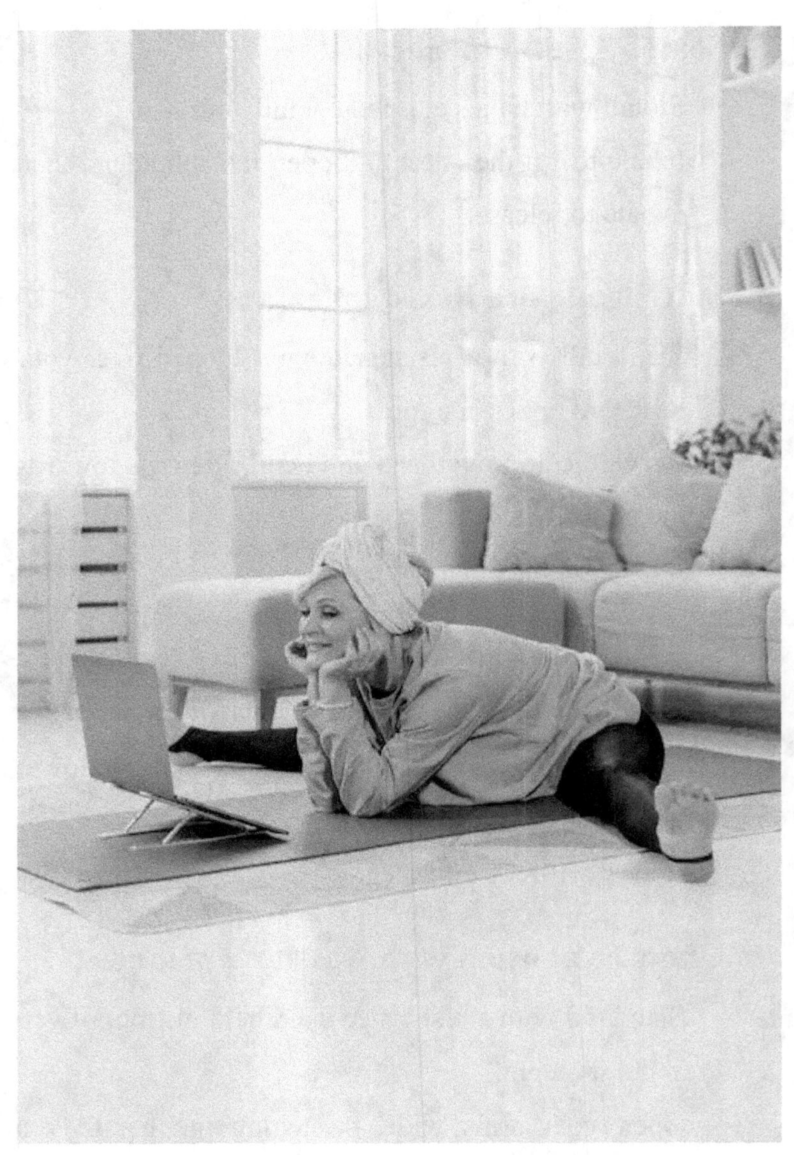

CONCLUSION

In conclusion, Pilates for seniors is a highly beneficial and transformative exercise regimen that offers a multitude of advantages for older adults. This gentle yet effective form of exercise focuses on core strength, flexibility, balance, and body awareness, catering to the unique needs and limitations of senior individuals.

Throughout this book, we have explored the numerous benefits that Pilates can bring to the lives of seniors, both physically and mentally.

First and foremost, Pilates promotes improved core strength, which plays a crucial role in supporting the spine and maintaining proper posture. As seniors age, issues with back pain and reduced stability become more common, making Pilates an ideal exercise to address these concerns.

The emphasis on core engagement during Pilates movements helps seniors build a strong foundation for everyday activities and enhances their overall physical functionality.

Furthermore, Pilates fosters enhanced flexibility, which is essential for maintaining a full range of motion in the joints and preventing stiffness and discomfort.

Seniors often face challenges with reduced flexibility, making Pilates' stretching exercises particularly valuable in promoting suppleness and joint health.

With increased flexibility, seniors can enjoy improved mobility, making it easier to engage in daily tasks and activities.

Balance and coordination are vital components of healthy aging, and Pilates addresses these areas as well. Many Pilates exercises involve performing movements while balancing on unstable surfaces, such as a stability ball or one leg, which helps seniors strengthen their balance and coordination skills.

This increased stability reduces the risk of falls, which can be a significant concern for older adults.

Pilates also contributes to improved bone density, a critical factor in preventing osteoporosis, a condition that weakens bones and makes them more prone to fractures.

Weight-bearing exercises, such as certain Pilates movements, help stimulate bone growth and maintenance, promoting better bone health and reducing the risk of fractures in seniors.

The mental benefits of Pilates for seniors should not be overlooked. The practice encourages mindfulness and body awareness, promoting a stronger mind-body connection. This heightened awareness helps seniors focus on their breath and movements, leading to reduced stress levels and enhanced mental well-being.

Additionally, Pilates classes provide a social outlet for seniors, fostering a sense of community and companionship, which is crucial for combating feelings of loneliness and isolation.

Throughout this book, we have also presented a comprehensive 14-day Pilates meal plan, highlighting the significance of combining a balanced diet with regular Pilates practice for optimal health. Proper nutrition complements the physical and mental benefits of Pilates, ensuring seniors have the energy and nutrients necessary for their bodies to function optimally.

In conclusion, Pilates for seniors is a versatile and inclusive exercise regimen that can significantly improve the quality of life for older adults. Its gentle yet effective nature makes it accessible to individuals of various fitness levels and accommodates the unique needs and limitations that come with aging.

By incorporating Pilates into their daily routines, seniors can enjoy a multitude of benefits, including increased core strength, enhanced flexibility, improved balance and coordination, better bone health, reduced stress levels, and a greater sense of community.

As the aging population continues to grow, it is crucial to emphasize the importance of maintaining a healthy and active lifestyle. Pilates offers seniors a safe and enjoyable way to stay physically and mentally fit, supporting their overall well-being and enabling them to lead fulfilling and vibrant lives as they embrace the golden years.

With the guidance of qualified instructors and a commitment to consistent practice, seniors can unlock the full potential of Pilates and reap the numerous rewards it has to offer.